The Magic of Sugar Cane

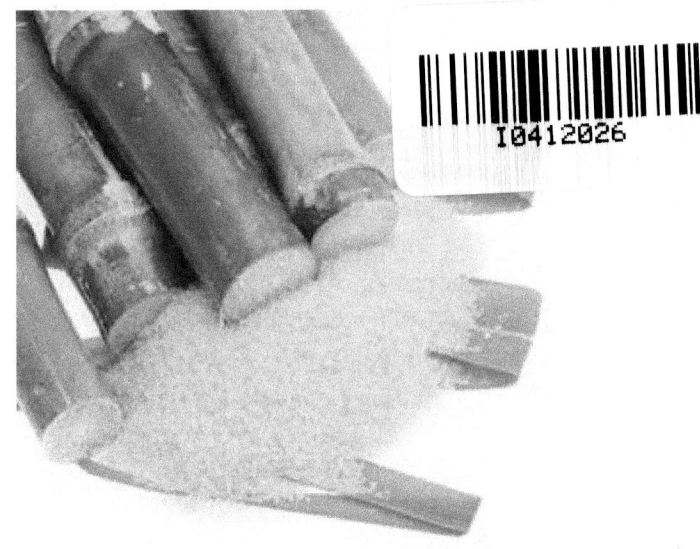

Health Learning Series

Dueep Jyot Singh

Mendon Cottage Books

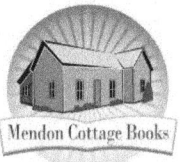

JD-Biz Publishing

All Rights Reserved.

Disclaimer

The information is this book is provided for informational purposes only. It is not intended to be used and medical advice or a substitute for proper medical treatment by a qualified health care provider. The information is believed to be accurate as presented based on research by the author.

The contents have not been evaluated by the U.S. Food and Drug Administration or any other Government or Health Organization and the contents in this book are not to be used to treat cure or prevent disease.

The author or publisher is not responsible for the use or safety of any diet, procedure or treatment mentioned in this book. The author or publisher is not responsible for errors or omissions that may exist.

Warning

The Book is for informational purposes only and before taking on any diet, treatment or medical procedure, it is recommended to consult with your primary health care provider.

Our books are available at

1. Amazon.com
2. Barnes and Noble
3. Itunes
4. Kobo
5. Smashwords
6. Google Play Books

Table of Contents

Introduction

Just imagine that you were living in Greece, Persia, or anywhere else in Southeast Asia, 3000 years ago and walking in a market garden. You would find plenty of gardeners selling you a "wonderful stick which has juice sweeter than honey." The sweetmeats that you ate would have been flavored with molasses or brown sugar, extracted from the juice from this "stick". It is supposed to have been domesticated in 6000 BC somewhere in New Guinea.

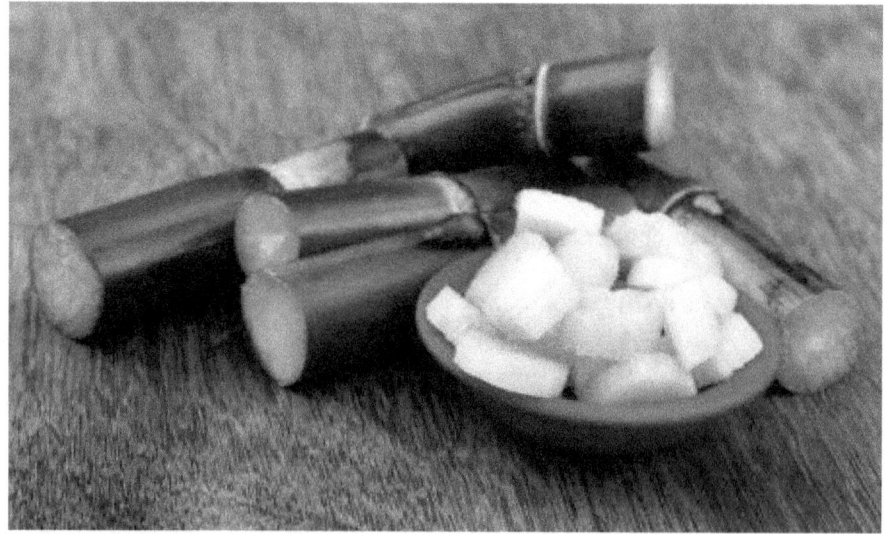

Peeled sugarcane is normally cut into bite sized chunks for future chewing. The left door fiber is then used as a fertilizer or as animal feed.

The Greeks and the Persians were not the only ones in ancient times who knew all about the magic of the sweet juice extracted from that long stout and fibrous jointed stalks anywhere between 3 – 6 m in height. This is a plant indigenous to Southeast and South Asia from where it spread all over the world to spread sweetness and joy no pun intended. It was marketed extensively all over the then known world under the excellent PR of "the reeds which are going to give you honey without any honeybees."

We know this juicy and succulent stick as sugarcane. It belongs to the family of grasses growing in tropical regions and temperate regions, where it is still the basis of the economy of many countries where it is grown in large quantities in sugarcane plantations.

These sugarcane plantations are spread globally, especially in the Caribbean regions, China, Mexico, the Indian subcontinent and Thailand. Christopher Columbus is supposed to have brought sugarcane to the Caribbean during one of his trips when he landed in Haiti and Dominica.

 The largest producer of sugarcane in the world is Brazil. Apart from the sugar production from this juice, Brazil also produces ethanol on a very large industrial scale from fermented juice. 26,000,000 ha produce 1.8 4,000,000,000 tons of sugarcane globally and annually.

Juice is not the only item which can be extracted from sugarcane. That "demon rum" is made from sugarcane, as are other fermented drinks like cachaça, bagasse and falernum.

The left over products after the extraction of juice are molasses, brown sugar [and we are not talking about South America's other popular product, also known as brown sugar in drug circles...] and jaggery.

Jaggery is the Indian equivalent of molasses, which is sold in a solidified form often with dried fruit embedded in it. This is also known as "gur" and is made by the evaporation of the juice till you get a brown sludge. This is then cooled in buckets, broken up into dark brown to light brown chunks, and then sold openly in the open-air markets of India.

Gur is normally used as a sugar substitute in many parts of India to sweeten tea, sweets, traditional sweetmeats and desserts.

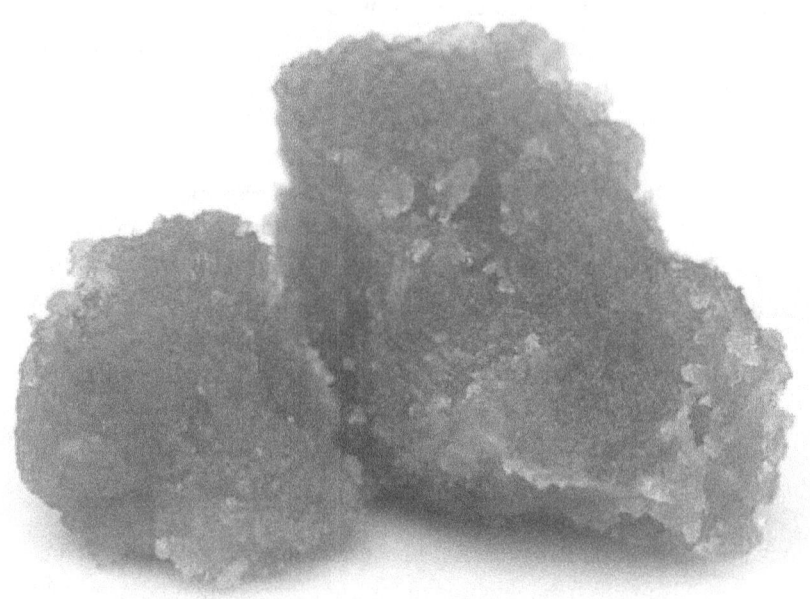

Along with giving your teeth plenty of dental exercise, when you chew on the sugarcane, the reeds of the sugarcane are used traditionally for thatching purposes. They are also useful in making floor mats and sunscreens. In Indonesian cuisine, the young sugarcane inflorescence is normally toasted, steamed or eaten raw.

Sugarcane plantations have been the backbone of many economies in the 17th, 18th and 19th century. Any person who irritated his straight-laced family members or even transgressed against the rules of society was immediately shipped off to learn How to Become a Man and get to know all about responsibility by overseeing the family plantations in the Caribbean regions, the Pacific, South America or in India.

It is a historically known fact that political offenders and criminals were "transported" as human slaves to work in the sugarcane fields of the Caribbean, in the 17th and 18th century from Europe.

This very important cash crop needed to be grown by only experienced growers. That is because it is very vulnerable to disease, insects, and the climate. You also need special tropical weather and soil to get a good sugarcane harvest. That means you would not be getting your 70 tons of sugarcane harvest per hectare, at that time. Thankfully modern farming know-how and advanced scientific technology gives us a yield of up to 180 tons per hectare depending on the crop and farming management techniques, we can put in use today.

Apart from this, one tropical typhoon was quite enough to bankrupt plantations and that is the reason why sugar was a luxury item in 17 century Europe.Sugarcane juice was made into molasses in the Caribbean and taken to Europe. It was than either made into rum or sold in the market as sugar.

No wonder the economies of Haiti, Barbados, Mauritius, Trinidad, Jamaica, Guadeloupe, and other islands in the sun rely heavily on sugarcane even today.

Cultivating Sugarcane

Sugarcane is traditionally cultivated in sub tropic, temperate and tropical regions of the world where you can get plenty of sun, air and water. You need anywhere between six – eight months of water every year, which can either be obtained through irrigation or through natural rainfall. No wonder so many tropical regions in the world where it rains all the time benefits from a good sugarcane crop.

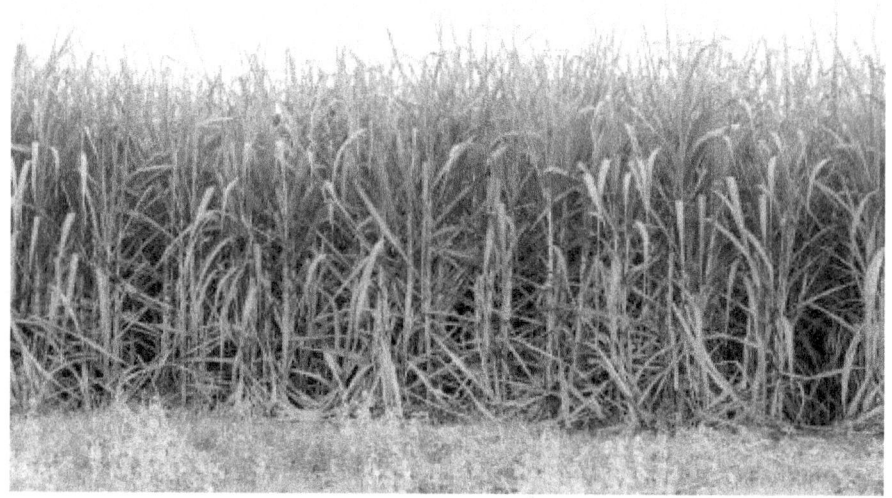

Sugarcane does not like cold weather or heights more than 1600 m, but this is only in places near the equator. The soil has to be very fertile and moist. Waterlogging in your sugarcane field is going to cause the rotting crop. Sorry if you have plenty of sunshine and plenty of water, you are going to get lots of sugarcane, as seen in Egypt and in other parts of Africa.

Sugarcanes normally grow from sugarcane cuttings, even though you can grow them from seeds if you have the time, inclination and energy to do so.

Every cutting should have on sugarcane plant bud. These cuttings are hand planted traditionally. After every harvest, every cane stalk is going to send out brand-new and fresh stalks. These are now called ratoons.

You are going to have the best harvest for the first four years. Subsequent years, to 10 years is going to lessen the harvest from the ratoons and you may want to replant a fresh new sugarcane crop.

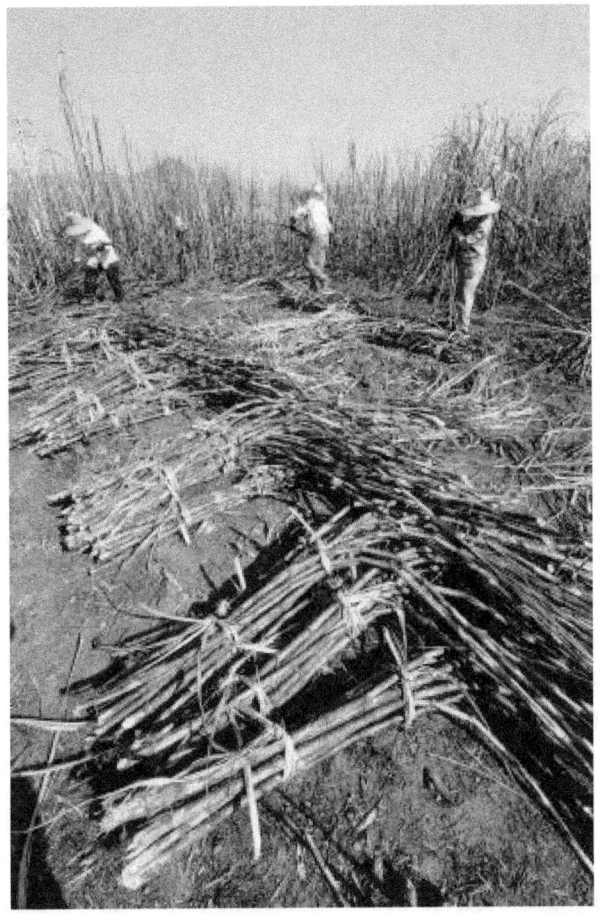

Your sugarcane harvest is going to be done either traditionally through cutting by hand. If the field is larger it is done mechanically. Hand harvesting is normally done in many parts of the world even today, where you do not have advanced technological development and the small size of the field does not justify the buying of an expensive harvesting machine.

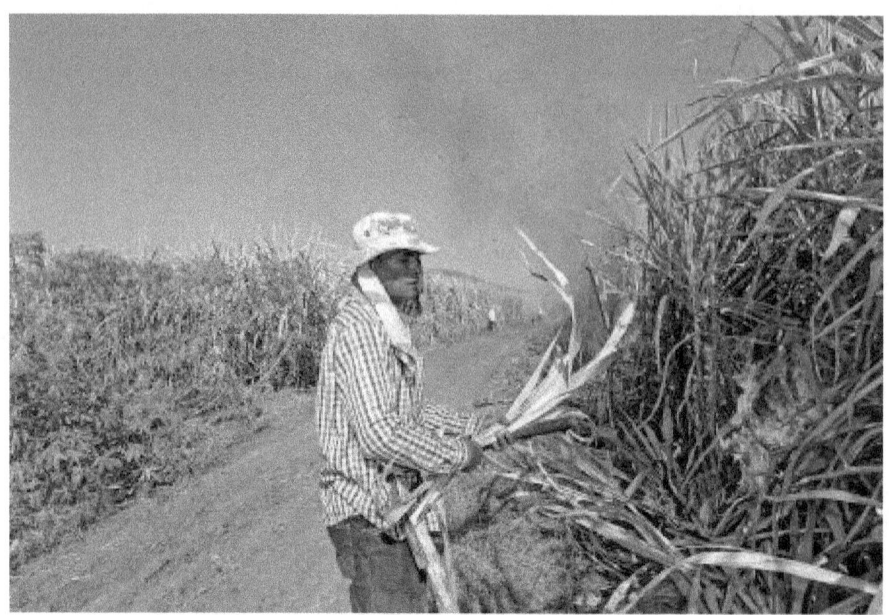

Setting Fire to the Fields is the first step before sugarcane harvesting.

Harvesting is done by setting the field on fire so that any snakes lurking in the dry leaves have enough time to disappear. This fire is not going to affect the roots and the stalks of the plants.

After that the harvesters enter the field to cut the sugarcane, either with machetes or with sugarcane knives. The cane is cut as near to the ground as possible. A really experienced harvester is capable of harvesting about 1000 pounds of sugarcane, in one hour!

The harvested sugarcane should be processed immediately because if it is left to itself, the sugar content is going to lessen. Mechanical harvesting may also cause some damage to the plant, which causes lessening of this sugar content. The leaves are left in the field, so that they can decompose as mulch after the harvesting is done.

Making Molasses

The traditional way of extracting sugarcane juice, and then heating it in a number of utensils in order to get a concentrated sugar form is still being followed in many parts of the world today.

I remember my grandmother telling me of sugarcane growers in her part of the country extracting sugarcane juice from freshly harvested cane by the side of the road going to places of pilgrimage. Every pilgrim going on this holy journey would be stopped by those farmers and given tall glasses of sugarcane juice to refresh themselves and quench their thirst.

I was under the impression that this idea of hospitality had gone with the 20th century, but a decade ago, I and my cousin along with a couple of aunts were driving down a village road on our way to one of our historical religious places. On our way back, we were stopped by farmers, who not only gave us fresh sugarcane juice to drink, but also gave my aunt and cousin a couple of pounds of freshly made hot brown sugar to take back to the US with them!

When my aunt offered them payment for the sugar, they immediately touched their ears, and shook their heads. In no manner were they going to take even one red cent from pilgrims, visiting holy places. According to them, they were gaining good Karma by quenching the thirst of all those who passed on the road and gaining their good wishes and blessings.

I do not know whether this tradition is being followed in other parts of the world, but I found it very heartwarming and pleasant.

There are three products which you are going to get when you extract juice from the sugarcane. First of all, you are going to get the bagasse, which is the dry sugarcane fiber residue from which all the juice has been extracted. The heated juice is going to concentrate into powdery brown sugar or solid molasses form depending on how much heating you have subjected it to. After that you are going to get filtercake.

In many parts of the world, the bagasse is normally used as a feed for cattle. It is also an excellent fuel and a mulch for your farmyard. Paper producing enterprises use bagasse, as well as other tree products to produce paper and other paper related products.

This bagasse also used as a fuel to stoke the boilers, when sugar is being made from the juice. The filter cake is totally dry and is an excellent fertilizer, and a supplement for feeding animals.

Molasses in the USA, takes the form of either molasses syrup or the stronger Blackstrap. Sugarcane growing in the USA is done in the Louisiana areas, where Blackstrap is very commonly used in traditional cuisine, or sold as a dietary supplement. They are also used as animal feed ingredients, or to make rum.

Many of the molasses products which you buy in the market today are going to be mixed with invert sugars, corn syrup or Maple syrup. So if you want pure Molasses, you need to visit a sugarcane plantation or a sugar mill.

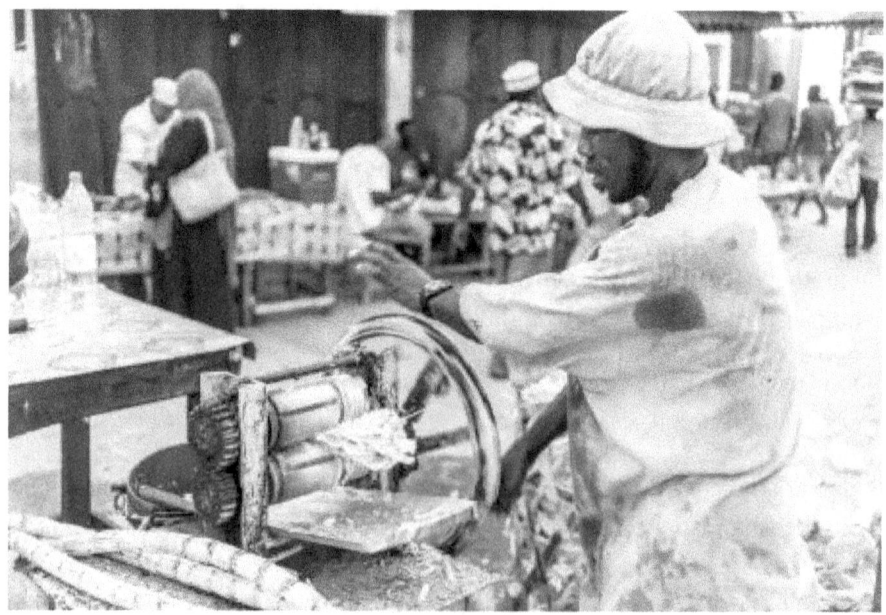

This Traditional Press is still in use all over the world.

In many parts of Southeast Asia, fresh sugarcane juice is always drunk by anyone working in the hot sun to prevent dehydration. This juice is extracted by a hand cranked press or mill. A little bit of lemon and ginger is added to it, and sometimes one also adds black salt, pepper, pieces of ice and mint to this brimming glass of sugarcane juice.

Sugarcane syrup was the first traditional choice as a sweetener in the USA, by manufacturers who were making sugar-based products, but they have now changed to an unhealthy product – corn syrup with a very high fructose level, because it is less costly and expensive. So the soft drinks you had before, flavored with sugarcane syrup is now flavored with harmful high fructose syrup made up of corn.

Crystallized cane sugar is known as rock candy all over the world. In the same manner, solid pieces of sugarcane juice, with lots of fructose and sucrose is a staple food in Central and South America. It is known as Panela. Also sugarcane juice is refined and made into a flour in the Caribbean, Argentina and other South American countries. This is known as papelón and Rapadura.

Sugarcane juice is also used to prevent sunstroke and heat stroke in tropical countries. Plenty of juice throughout summer is going to keep your kidneys functioning in a healthy manner. People suffering from diabetes should avoid sugarcane products and sugarcane juice.

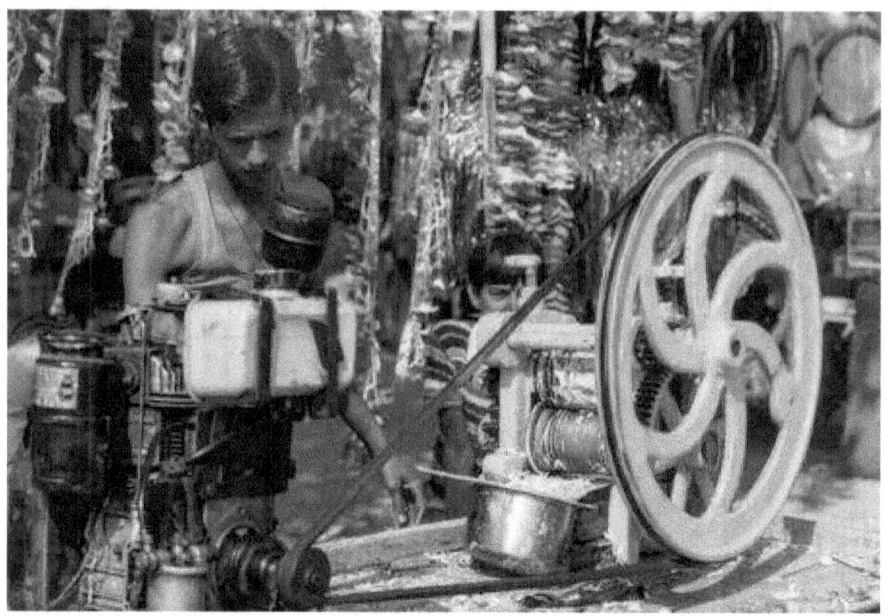

Sugarcane Juice on the road. Unhygienic, but a part of the summer scene in the Indian subcontinent. The juice is extracted in the metal utensil into which a lemon has already been squeezed.

Sugarcane for Health

Sugarcane, especially sugarcane juice and sugarcane molasses has long been used in ancient medicine to treat a number of ailments. This is because it has a number of important nutrients, which can help cure your problems.

Kidney Stone Treatment

You don't need to suffer from pain related to kidney stones if you have sugarcane around you.

In Ancient Southeast Asian medicine sugarcane juice has been the best way by which kidney stones were eliminated from the system. So if you are suffering from any sort of kidney stones, pick up a sugarcane cane.

Either bite into it and chew the bite sized pieces, or have as many glasses of sugarcane, you can manage to get down during the day. You are soon going to find that your system clears up and the stones are going to break up into small pieces of their own volition. They are going to then get eliminated naturally with the other toxic wastes of your body through your elimination system.

Jaundice

Sugarcane juice is the traditional natural cure for jaundice, down the ages in Asia. I remember my younger brother suffering from jaundice, one terrible summer. The doctors filled him up with drugs which did not seem to have any visible effect on his health. In fact, he started to weaken until we came down to our ancestral village for our annual holidays.

The elders of the village took one look at him and asked my father details about the one eyed burg place to which he had been transferred where nobody could get fresh sugarcane. If he had sense, he would have fed the poor ailing lad fresh sugarcane juice, instead of putting his son's health in the hands of those people practicing medicine.

Three glasses of fresh sugarcane juice along with one sugarcane bitten and chewed early in the morning and my brother was cured within a week. We did not know at that time that there was even another more powerful ingredient which was also taken with sugarcane in order to lessen the curing time – this is ordinary barley water. Drinking barley water instead of ordinary water would have helped cure him even faster.

Here is a video about how barley water is being made as a probiotic drink and food supplement in today's world. There was once a time when barley water was used extensively as invalid food and food for people with dedicated digestive systems. But as it is a cereal, take full benefit of it.

https://www.youtube.com/watch?v=BnyemRTrJZc

If you do not suffer from jaundice and want to drink barley water as a health drink, here is another amusing URL with extras added in your barley water.

http://www.happyjuicer.com/make-barley-water.aspx

It is said traditionally about the sugarcane that people as thin as a stick could grow healthy and begin to put on weight, by eating sugarcane after their meals. The answer is simple. The sugarcane juice is an excellent digestive. It also gives energy to the body because of its sucrose content. The system tones up and you are going to find yourself healthier.

In the 19 century when the Britishers ruled over the Indian subcontinent, they were subjected to heat stroke, as well as cholera every year with the coming of the rains. But they did not believe in traditional medicine, because according to them, that was barbaric and heathen knowledge and so they died like flies in their shoes.

However, the natives protected themselves by drinking fresh sugarcane juice with ginger, lemon juice and red pepper. This was the traditionally accepted way in which one could protect oneself from cholera, or any other waterborne diseases.

Well, here is my scientific explanation for how this happened. The term is waterborne. Cholera was spread through drinking infected and tainted water, but if a person drank sugarcane juice instead of infected water, the chances were great that he would not suffer from cholera. QED.

The Healthy Use of Jaggery

Jaggery or the Indian solid molasses has long been used in ancient medicine to make up medical remedies with herbs added to the sugarcane sugar. In India, molasses are not as concentrated as jaggery and is known as Khand. Jaggery is known as gud/gur , and it tastes just like its name, really good in sweetmeats.

Here is a traditional sciatica cure for all those people who suffer from this impossible problem in the winter, or whenever the weather is wet and inclement.

Sciatica Cure

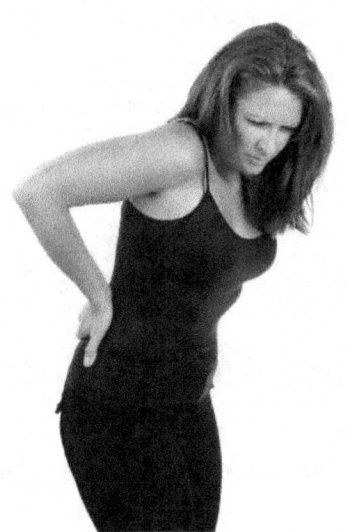

This is a surefire recipe for the cure of sciatica. So if you find yourself going out in all weathers, and find yourself susceptible to shooting pain in your legs, make up this recipe right now.

Take equal amounts of red Alum[1] (white alum won't do) and Jaggery[2]. Jaggery is indigenous to the East, because it is even more concentrated than

---

[1] http://www.citycollegiate.com/alum.htm gives you more information about alum.

molasses. Molasses won't do either, tough luck. Heat the alum in a frying pan until it comes out white.

Now powder the jaggery, and mix it with the Alum with your fingers. Half a teaspoon morning and night with a glass full of milk for one month will cure you of that pain in the leg, permanently!

Curing Bronchitis

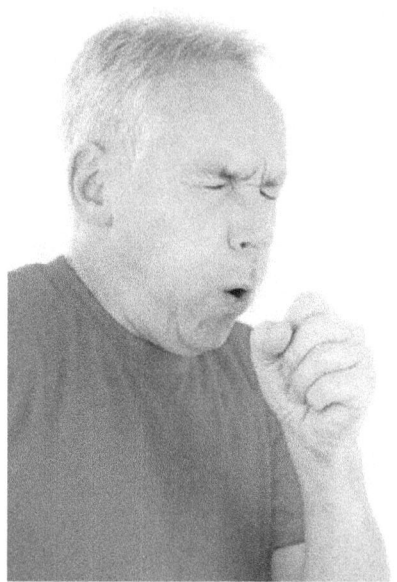

You can prevent as well as cure bronchitis by eating pieces of jaggery sprinkled with the large number of sesame seeds in the winter. In the same

---

[2] http://www.amazon.com/2-2-Lbs-Organic-Jaggery-Wholesome/dp/B009OJW5OW/ref=sr_1_1?ie=UTF8&qid=1423558874&sr=8-1&keywords=jaggery+gur

This is expensive, but like I said, it is pure and organic sugar made up of sugarcane and definitely better than chemically refined white sugar. You may also want to look for organic brown sugar on other sites in South America and in Southeast Asia. Look for panela , which is also known as gur.

manner, if you are prone to cough and cold in the winter, eat this mixture of jaggery and sesame whenever you can throughout the day. This is going to build up your internal resistance to external infections and attacks from diseases.

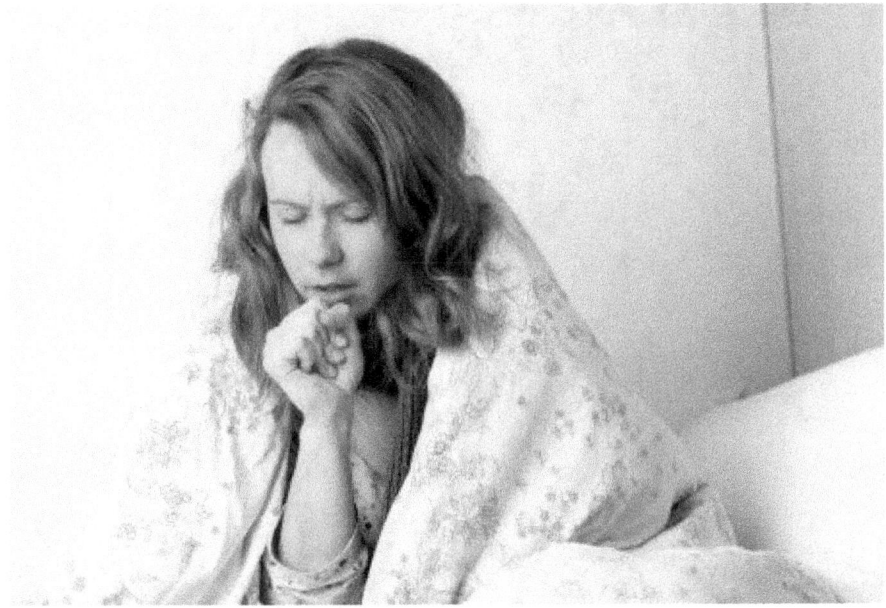

Let me give you my own bronchitis cure with the help of this jaggery. Add five peppercorns – ground lightly – and 1/8 teaspoon full of dried ginger to this mixture, when you are ready to chew it. Peppercorns are the best heat producing spices for winter and ginger is the ancient curative remedy for preventing coughs and colds in the winter, since ancient times.

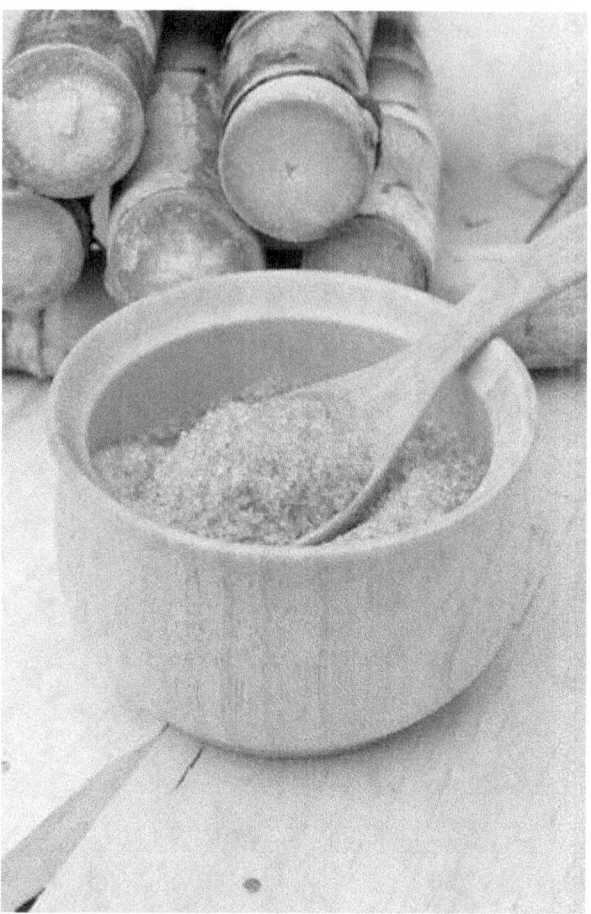

Curing Headaches

Now this is one cure which I have tried out myself, and found remarkably effective. I found myself suffering from tension headaches about five years ago, when I had a very high power and responsible job. And these waxed and waned as the sun rose and set.

You could call this auto suggestion because the moment I woke up, and I knew I had to go through a whole day, settling union disputes and management idiocies, Oh Someone Save Me...

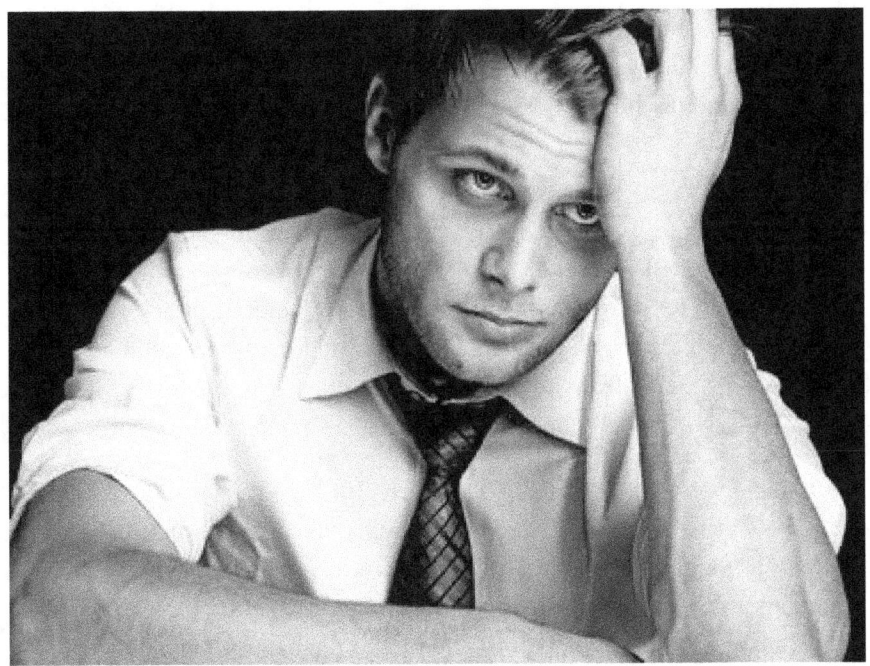

Tension headaches are very common among professionals under stress. Prevent and cure them by increasing your intake of molasses/jaggery.

One day I found myself with a very low sugar level,- which had an equally detrimental effect on my temper and patience-and I did not have anything sweet to pop into my mouth. But a colleague was celebrating some joyous occasion and had brought a box full of traditional sweets to the office. These sweets were made of molasses/brown sugar/jaggery.

So I had a couple of them and found to my surprise that my headache had begun melting away. I decided that it was just because everybody around me was behaving in a civilized manner and not shouting and creating tension for yours truly! But I soon found out that it was possibly because of the jaggery content in the sweetmeats.

That evening I went straight to my friendly neighborhood grocers shop and asked for pure organic sugar, one kg. "With or without dry fruit," He asked me. Dry fruit? In jaggery? Seems unusual. Anyway, the price difference between the ordinary variety and the dry fruit variety was rather a wee bit much, so I decided to buy half a pound of ordinary brown sugar

I began eating half a teaspoonful in yogurt for lunch and had half a teaspoonful of it in a glass full of milk in the afternoon.[3] , and surprisingly enough, I found my headaches vanishing away. [4]

Molasses as a Diuretic

A friend of mine told me that she was taking diuretics to get rid of all the toxins in her body. I was taken aback, because there are so many people out there who go in for unwanted medication ideas just because they have something remotely vague brewing in their mind. So as my friend equated the removal of toxins from her body with diuretics, she was dozing herself in a particularly nasty and potentially dangerous manner.

Do not you ever try anything like that ever. But if you do want to get rid of accumulated toxins, here is the natural way in which you can clear out your system. Take a glass full of hot milk. Add a teaspoonful of jaggery/molasses to it. Gulp it down. Do this twice a day and find your system clearing up miraculously. You may find yourself going to the bathroom a number of times when you take this treatment. Try this for three days.

When I told my friend to try this treatment instead of using diuretics, she

told me whether she could continue drinking hot milk and jaggery, because she had gotten addicted to that combination! And here is the answer. "Of course you can. You are getting healthy milk in you, under any pretext twice a day, are not you. So go right ahead."

---

[3] You can increase the quantity according to your taste and if you are not diabetic. I am not, but I just do not like the taste of anything sweet. You can also add this to your coffee or to your tea, which I did not because I do not drink these particular beverages at all.

[4] I have not – knock on wood – suffered from a headache since that magical day I resigned from that high tension high paying job in 2010. So apart from the healthy organic sugar, a relief from tension and stress could also have caused the cessation of headaches.

Constipation Cure

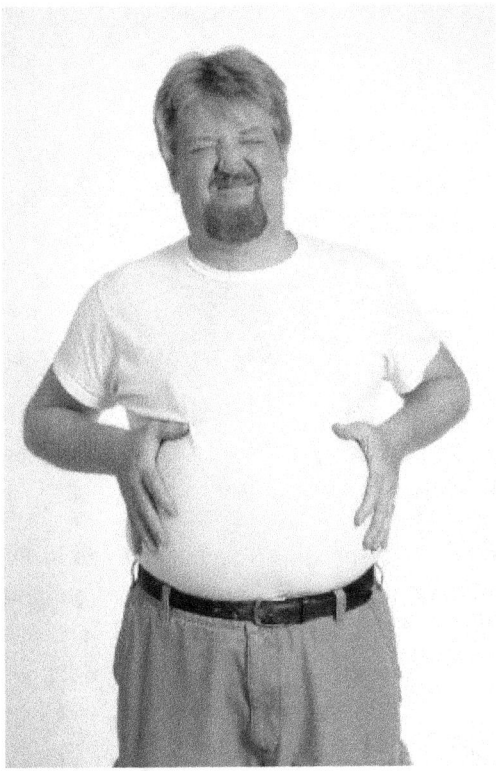

Apart from being an excellent diuretic, the hot milk and jaggery combination is excellent for people suffering from constipation. So instead of putting a spoonful of sugar in your milk, add a piece of jaggery. Stir well and drink down fast.

There is only one drawback of eating too much of jaggery. You are eating sugar in a highly concentrated form. So if you are prone to diabetes, do not touch it. Also, too much of jaggery eaten by children is supposed to produce "heat." That is why they are not fed any molasses or jaggery in the summer.

It is also not eaten in the rainy season when one is more prone to skin diseases. Too much of molasses in this weather could cause an outbreak of skin problems like boils and pimples.

Dyspepsia Cure

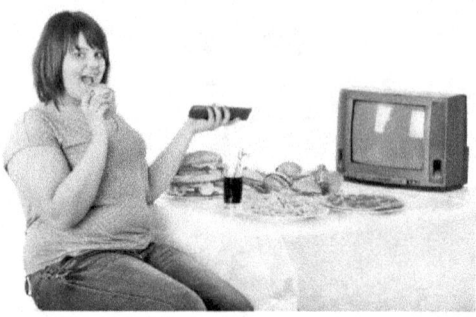

Eating Too Much and eating "unhealthy" food is going to cause stomach problems. Add jaggery/molasses to your daily diet to help digest all these huge meals.

If you are suffering from dyspepsia all you have to do is break off a piece of molasses/organic jaggery from its solid block after you have finished your meal. Chew with two mouthfuls of water. In many parts of the East meals are always ended with pieces of jaggery and water, even today. So 25 g of jaggery eaten after every meal is going to keep you free from dyspepsia and other stomach problems.

Also, this traditionally eaten piece of jaggery after every meal prevents you from suffering from flatulence while aiding in your digestive system.

Jaggery as a Rejuvenating Food

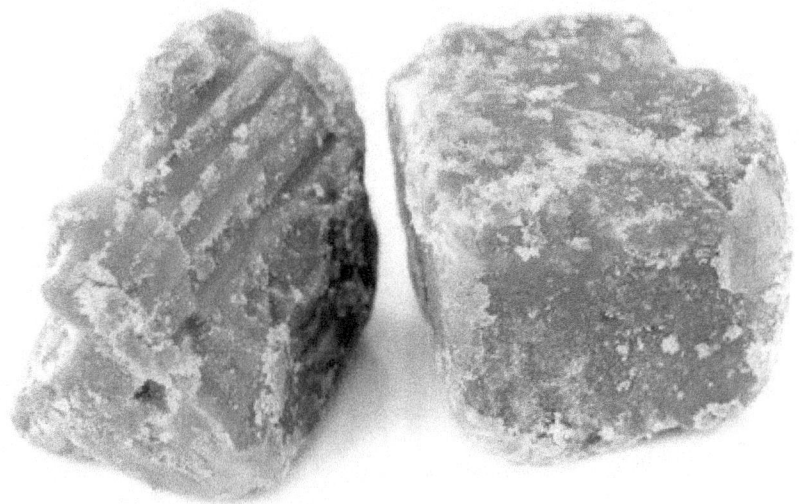

I once asked an experienced herbalist about the benefits of jaggery as a health food, especially to keep one more youthful and younger looking. He told me that the remedy was so simple that it was surprising that more people did not use it. All you had to do was drink a glass full of hot milk with jaggery, before going to sleep.

Not only would this help cure insomnia, but it would also keep your body warm, especially in the winters. You would not suffer any constipation. You would also not need to go to the bathroom at night, or suffer from dehydration, which woke you up in the middle of the night feeling so thirsty.

Molasses in Traditional Cuisine

Molasses Rice pudding

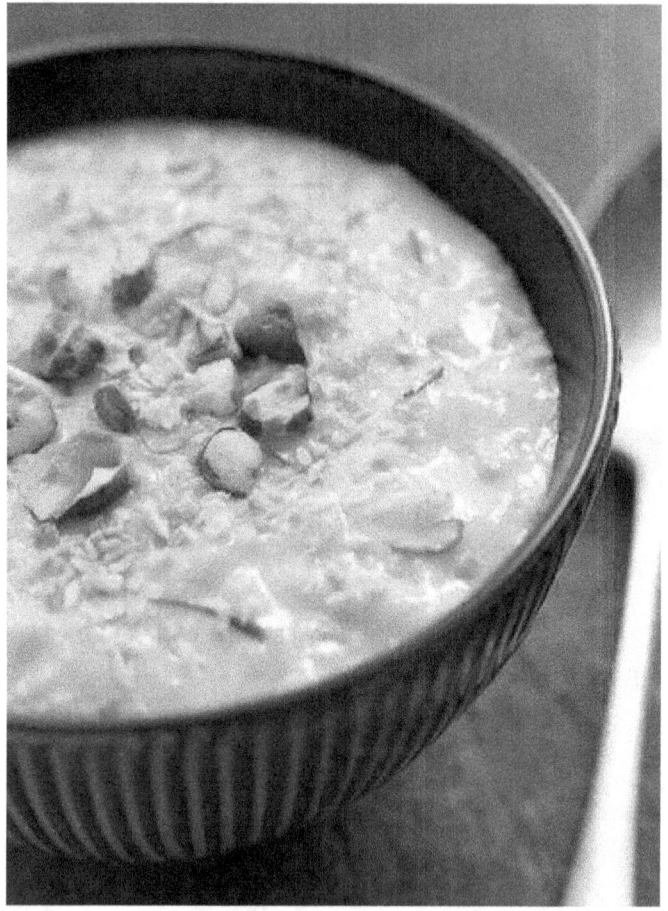

This is a traditional rice pudding, which is normally eaten as a popular dessert, or with the addition of saffron and dry fruit, as a popular festive dish on special occasions. Honey, molasses and jaggery were the usual ways in which people traditionally sweetened the sweet dishes down the ages. So is it a surprise that rice pudding is going to be made up of brown sugar or molasses.

For this you need 600 mL of milk, 30 grams of rice, three large chunks of jaggery, or six – 7 tablespoons of powdered molasses. This is according to taste. The rest of the items are optional and include dry fruits like a few raisins, a few launched almonds, 2 cardamoms crushed. A few drops of rose water or vanilla essence and a few pistachio nuts. You can also add your favorite dried fruit and nuts as desired.

Wash the rice and soak in water for 15 minutes. Boil the milk in a heavy pan. Add the rice, which has been strained, stir and allow to boil for a few minutes.

Then reduce to a low heat and allow to simmer. Stir it occasionally and then add all the spices – raisins, cardamoms and almonds.

When the milk is thick enough and the rice has been well cooked, add the molasses and raise the heat, stirring continuously to prevent sticking.

Remove from heat and mix in a few drops of rose water or essence. Put in a bowl and allow to cool in the refrigerator. Garnish with pistachio nuts and serve.

I normally eat this with a spoonful of fresh cream, swirled and spread on the cool surface, because I'm not a weight watcher. Guaranteed delicious and addictive. Also, you may find the rest of your family demanding the uppermost layer of the cold rice pudding. It is going to consist of a thick layer of rice pudding mixed with milk cream rising to the top. Also the cooked milk stuck to the sides of the pan, after the milk pudding has been poured out in its bowl is also very delicious, when scraped with a spoon and eaten straight from the pan.[5]

---

[5] Some hilarious memories, of childhood. I being top spoilt brat and bully of the family used to grab the saucepan after grandmother had finished making this rice pudding and begin scraping with my spoon without sharing any of those gleaned portions with my younger brother or with anyone else.

My grandmother once clicked her tongue and said, "well, they say that anyone who does not share the bounty of the cooking pan with other members of the family is going to have a totally wet and soggy wedding day. She is also going to suffer from lots of rain on every joyous occasion. "

Traditional Whole Wheat Bread

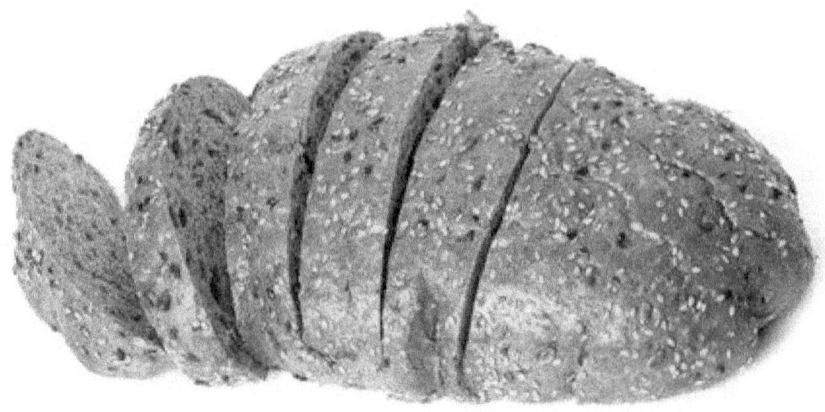

This bread has sesame seeds sprinkled on the top

For this you need 2 cups of scalded milk, 1/3 cups of molasses, 2 teaspoons full of salt, one tablespoonful of yeast, ¼ cup of warm water, 4 2/3 cups of whole wheat flour

Add the molasses to the milk. Let it cool to lukewarm. Dissolve yeast in the lukewarm water.

That made me think a little – just a little bit. Now I see, that it was really ancient psychology – the threat of rain on joyous occasions. But common sense [and greed] prevailed and I retorted that rainy wedding days, and so on could take care of themselves and they were too far in the future to be considered, but at the moment, I wanted to finish up all the cooked scrapings attached to the cooking pan.

Grandmother gave up. But I wonder how many people before me learned the lesson of sharing, with this threat hanging over them! Talk about the wisdom of the East!

Put all the liquids together. Add them as you keep stirring to the flour into which you have already mixed salt, beat well, and cover. Let the bread rise to double in bulk.

Knead again and turn into greased bread pan so that the pans are half full.

Allow to rise in a warm place until almost doubled in size. Bake at 400°F for about 15 minutes until it shrinks from the sides of the pan.

Butter the top a few minutes before removing from the oven.

Grandma's Molasses Candy

2 cups molasses, 1 cup sugar and one tablespoonful of vinegar.

Cook together until crunchy and brittle when dropped in cold water. Stir in a pinch of baking soda and 3 cups of chopped black walnuts. Pour into greased pan. Break into pieces, when cold.

Conclusion

You have now been introduced to the magic of sugarcane. Not only is this excellent for your health, but it is also easy to grow in your garden.

Here are some URLs, which you would like to watch, especially as they are so interesting.

This URL is about how you can grow sugarcane in your own yard.

https://www.youtube.com/watch?v=T8OP6Jzuzgw

I also found this URL put up by Tom Allen, on how to make molasses, really good viewing.

https://www.youtube.com/watch?v=qpbUdAcpA20

The traditional way of making molasses may be unknown to the younger generation, but it is still being practiced in many parts of the world. Even today, hand cranked machines are used to extract juice which is then boiled on open fires in open fields and in large metal pots.[6]

Also, this is also very informational, especially when one is talking about molasses as an organic fertilizer. You're going to use it, when you have plenty of molasses at hand and you can use it liberally in your garden. Why not, it is natural compost.

http://www.smilinggardener.com/organic-fertilizers/molasses-as-fertilizer

And for those people who enjoy cooking, here is the touch of the real South, on this URL.

http://www.brerrabbit.com/cooking-with-molasses/

I'm certain the traditional baked bean and molasses dish was very popular in our grandmother's day and y'all could be sure that it was finger lickin'

---

[6] Nobody bothers much about air pollution because that's the way it has been done down the ages…

good. In fact, before the Civil War, beans, pork and molasses seemed to be the staple diet of many people in the South. But then it is a really tasty combination,Suh! Also, Creole cooking in Louisiana traditionally uses plenty of molasses as an important kitchen ingredient while dishing up toothsome fare.

Peanut Brittle

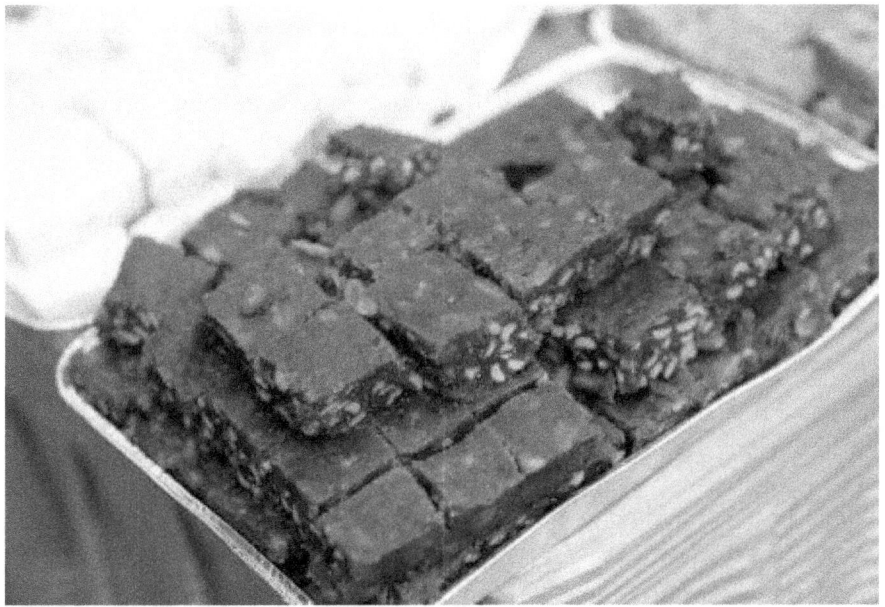

When I was a kid, this peanut brittle called a Chikki was very much in demand in our school canteen. It sold for an equivalent of less than half a cent per piece. [Those were the days my friend…] It still seems to be very popular on YouTube!

https://www.youtube.com/watch?v=vKnKQaj27bg

Seeing the instructions on this URL, I can see that this particular Brittle is universally popular. The instructions are given in English below the video, so switch the sound to mute and watch the video!

Live Long and Prosper!

Author Bio

Dueep Jyot Singh is a Management and IT Professional who managed to gather Postgraduate qualifications in Management and English and Degrees in Science, French and Education while pursuing different enjoyable career options like being an hospital administrator, IT,SEO and HRD Database Manager/ trainer, movie , radio and TV scriptwriter, theatre artiste and public speaker, lecturer in French, Marketing and Advertising, ex-Editor of Hearts On Fire (now known as Solstice) Books Missouri USA, advice columnist and cartoonist, publisher and Aviation School trainer, ex-moderator on Medico.in, banker, student councilor ,travelogue writer … among other things!

One fine morning, she decided that she had enough of killing herself by Degrees and went back to her first love -- writing. It's more enjoyable! She already has 48 published academic and 14 fiction- in- different- genre books under her belt.

When she is not designing websites or making Graphic design illustrations for clients , she is browsing through old bookshops hunting for treasures, of which she has an enviable collection – including R.L. Stevenson, O.Henry, Dornford Yates, Maurice Walsh, De Maupassant, Victor Hugo, Sapper, C.N. Williamson, "Bartimeus" and the crown of her collection- Dickens "The Old Curiosity Shop," and so on… Just call her "Renaissance Woman") - collecting herbal remedies, acting like Universal Helping Hand/Agony Aunt, or escaping to her dear mountains for a bit of exploring, collecting herbs and plants and trekking.

Check out some of the other JD-Biz Publishing books

Gardening Series on Amazon

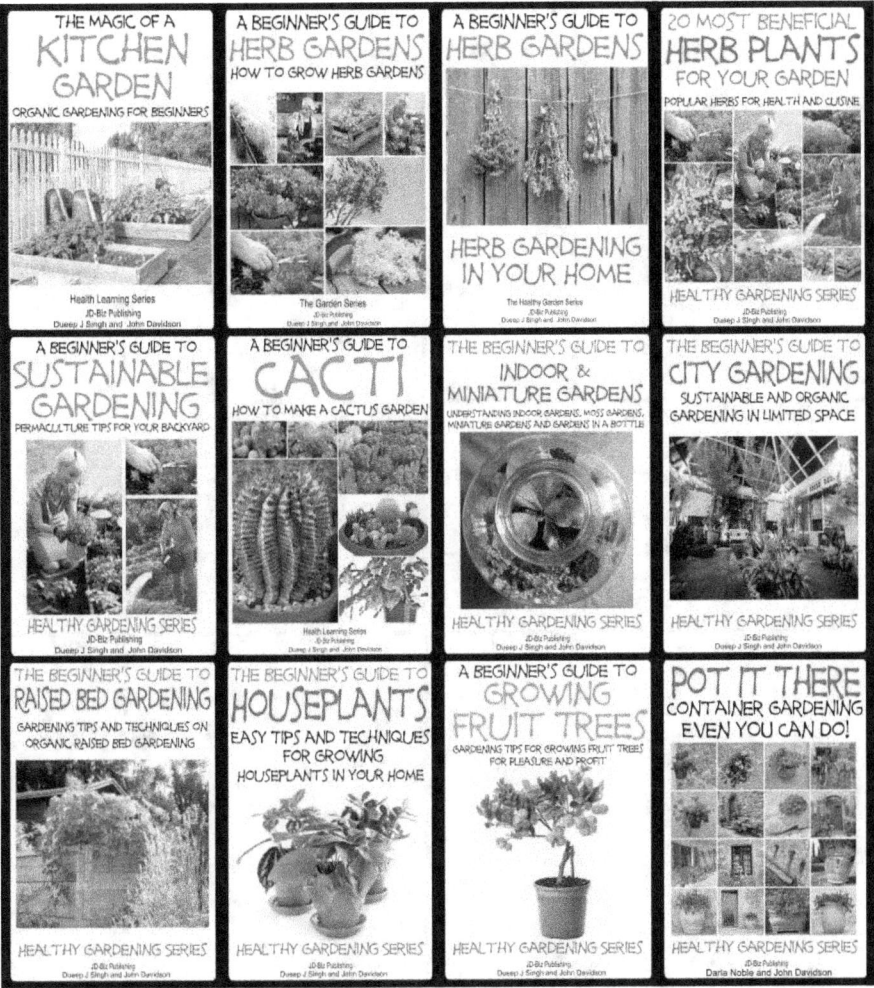

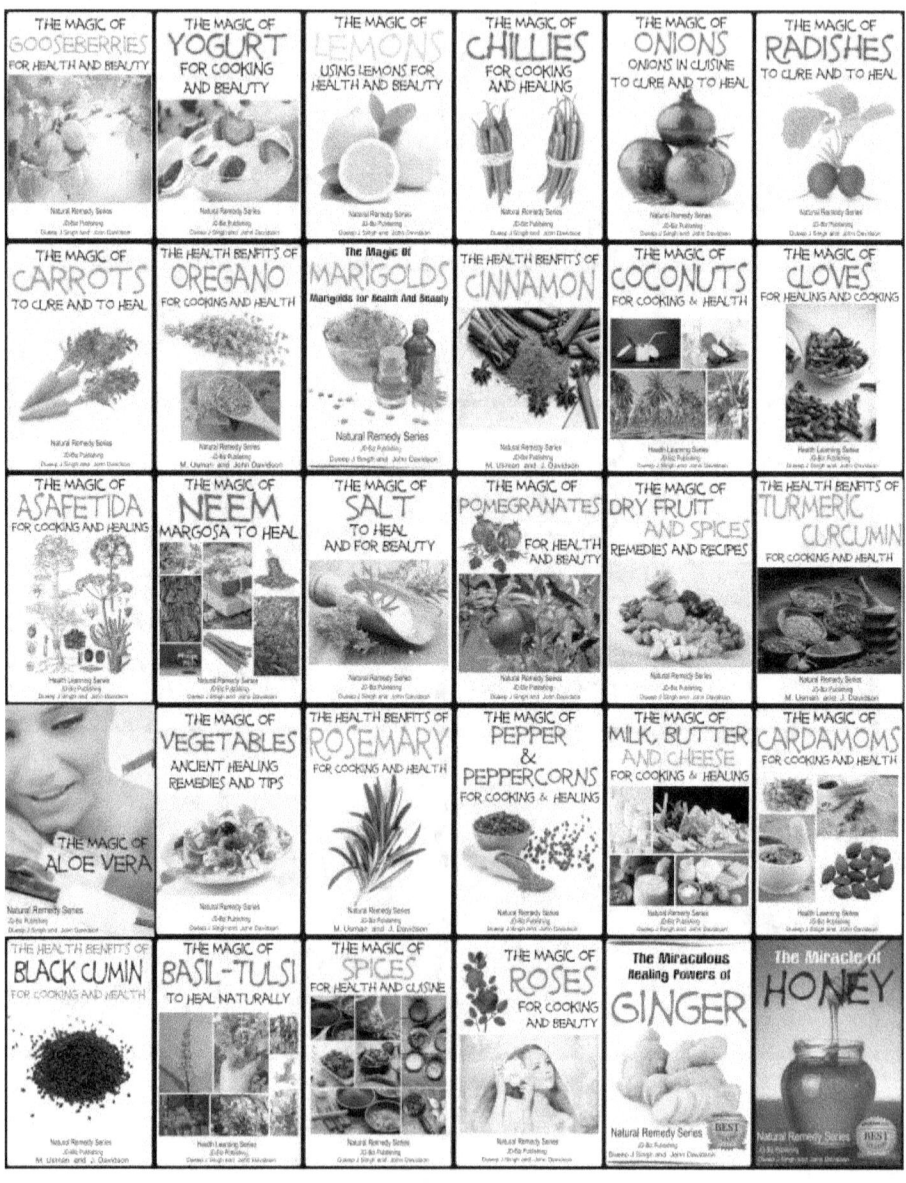

Country Life Books

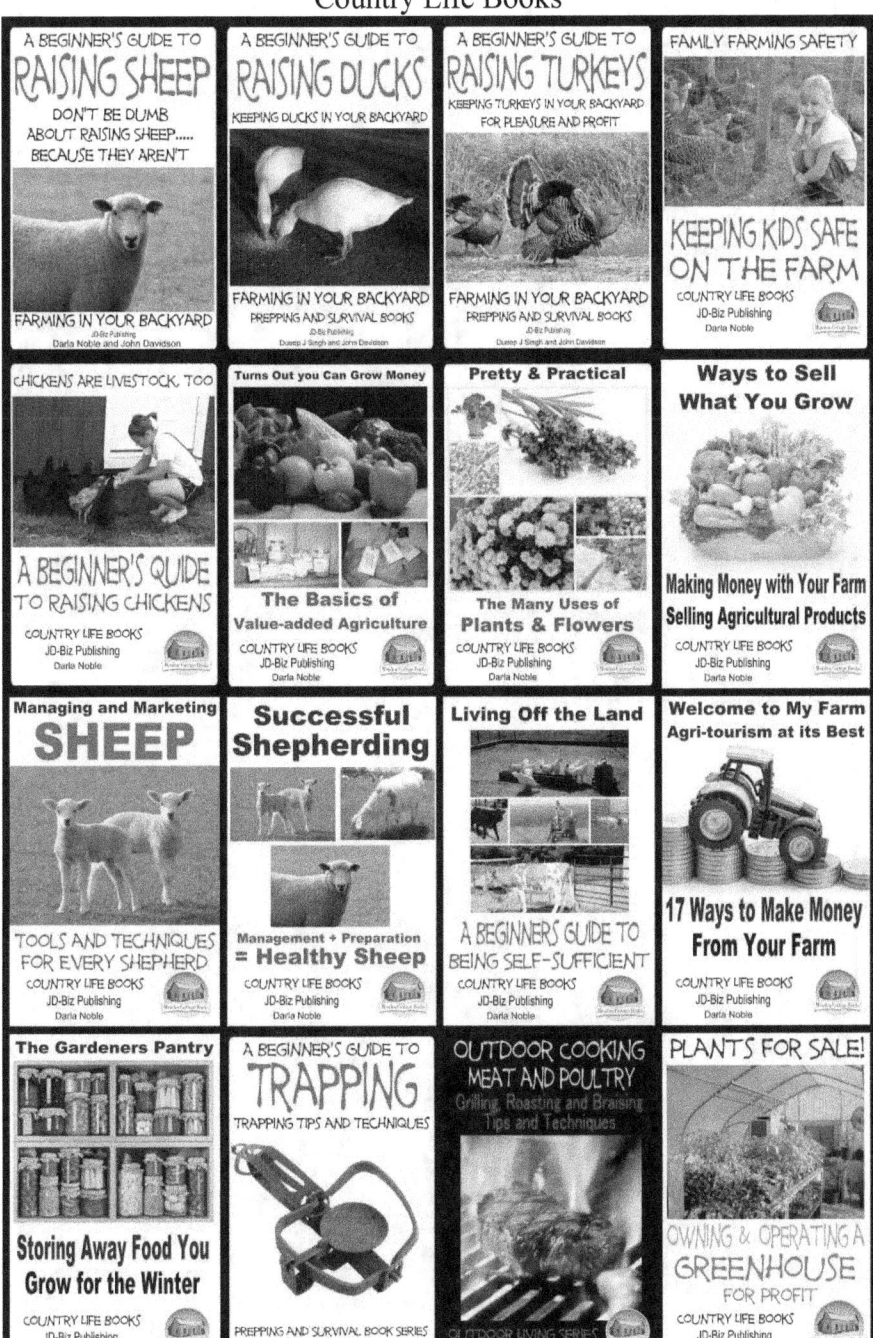

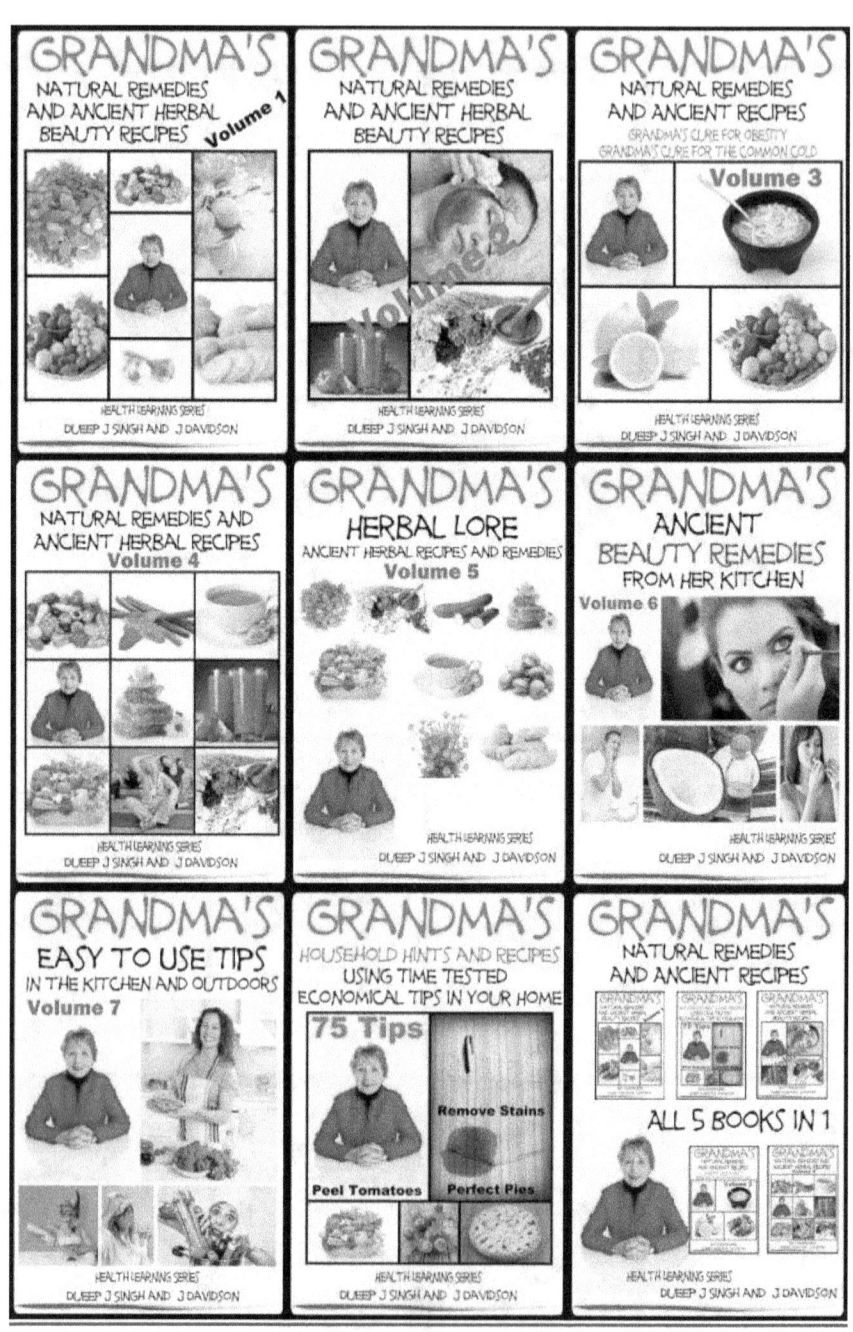

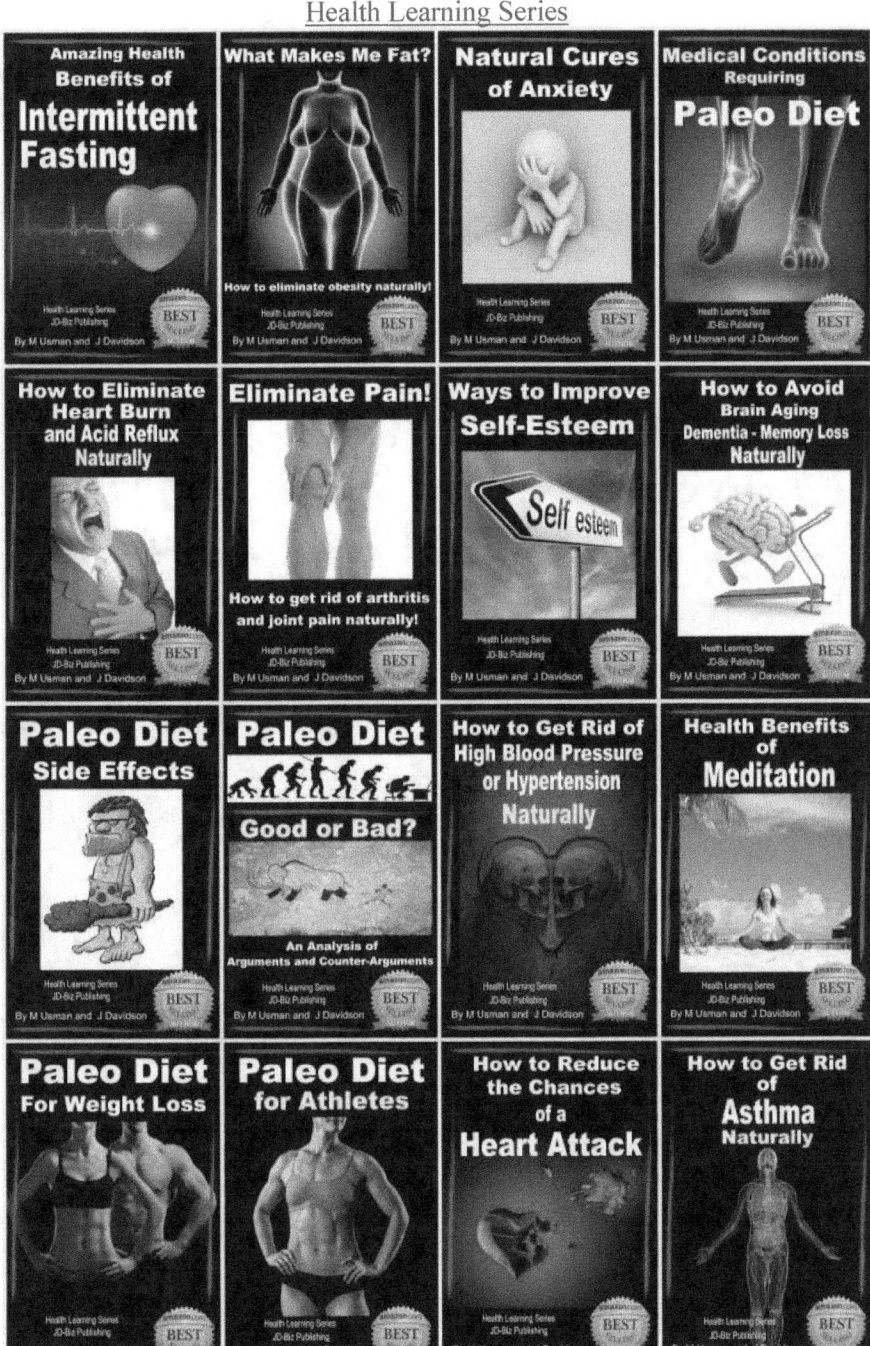

Amazing Animal Book Series

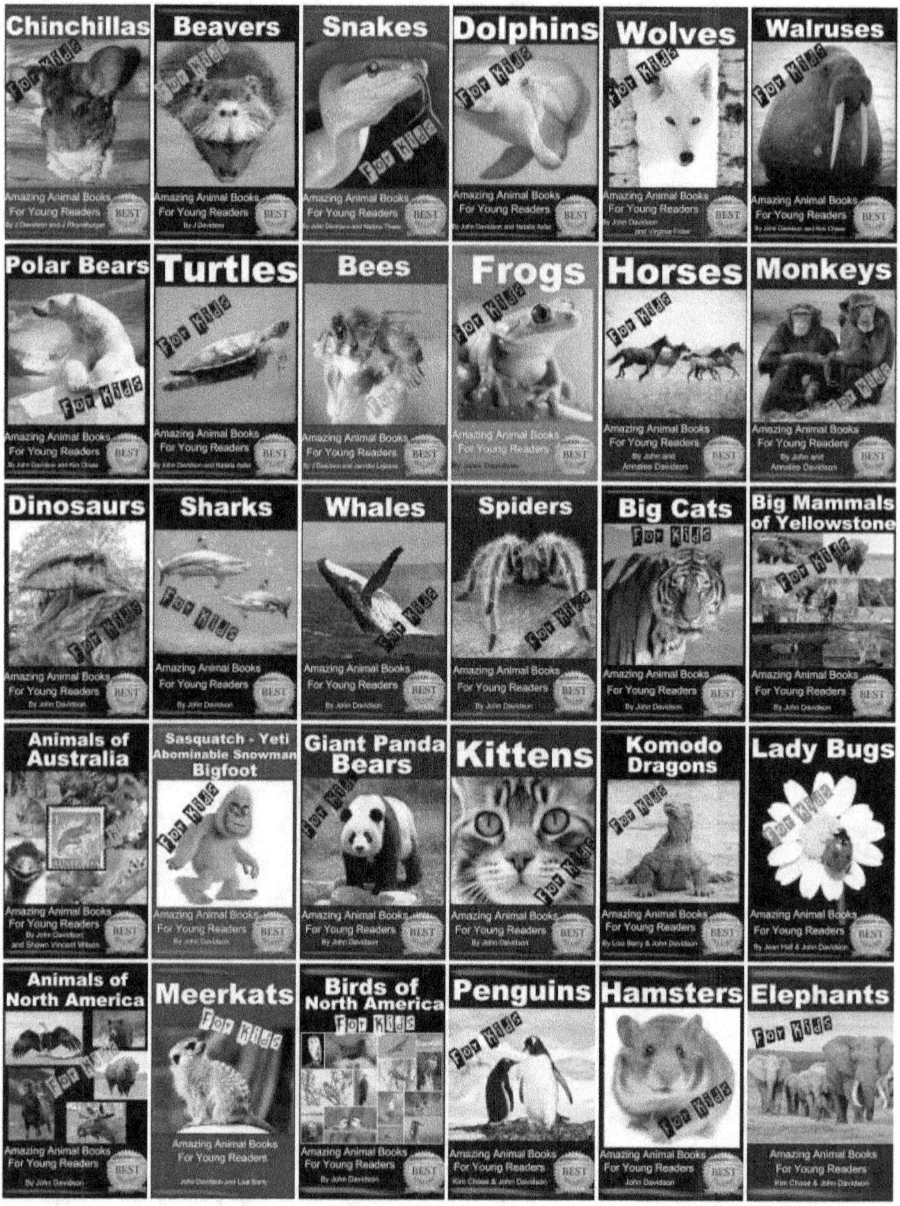

Learn To Draw Series

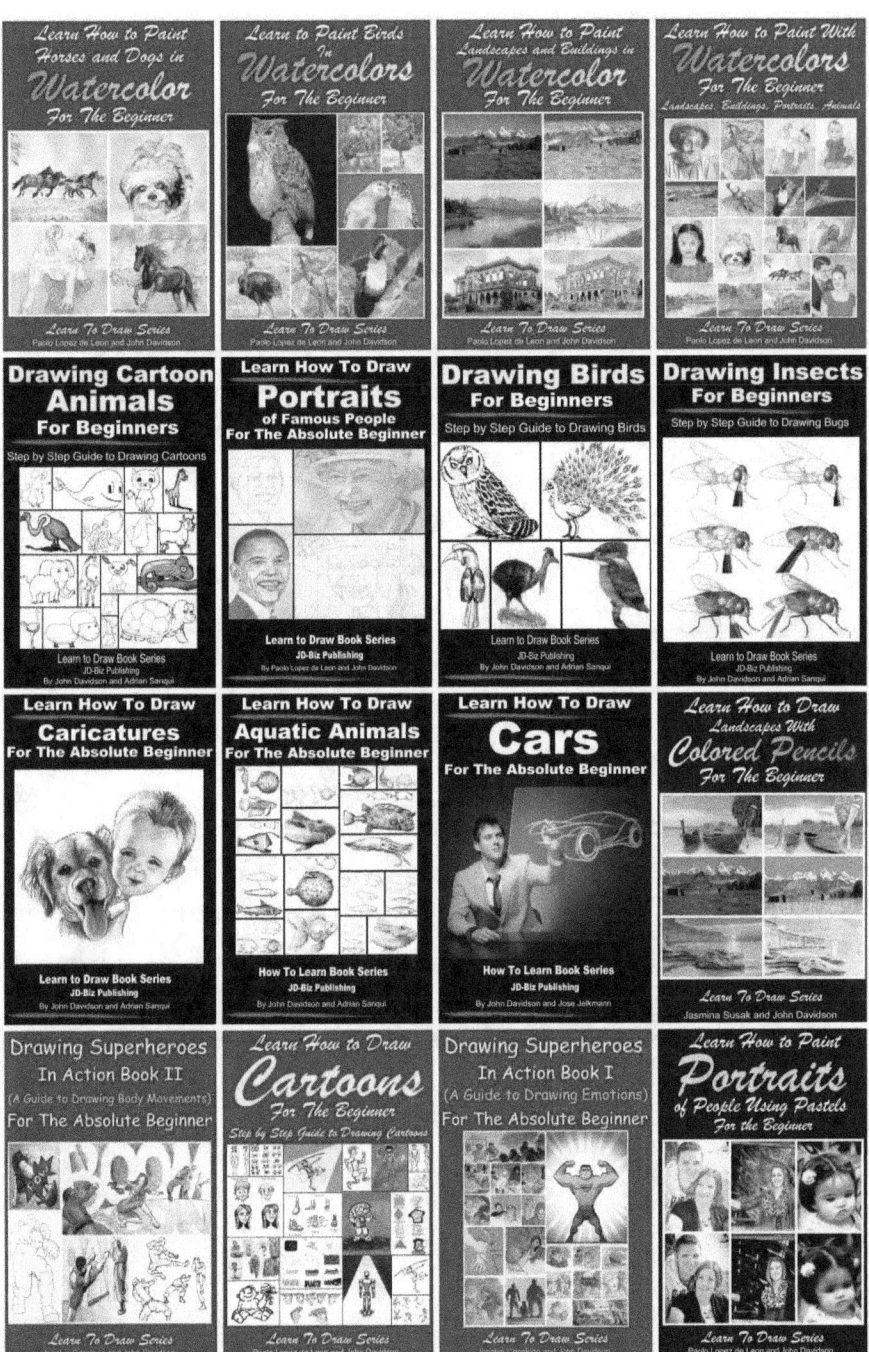

How to Build and Plan Books

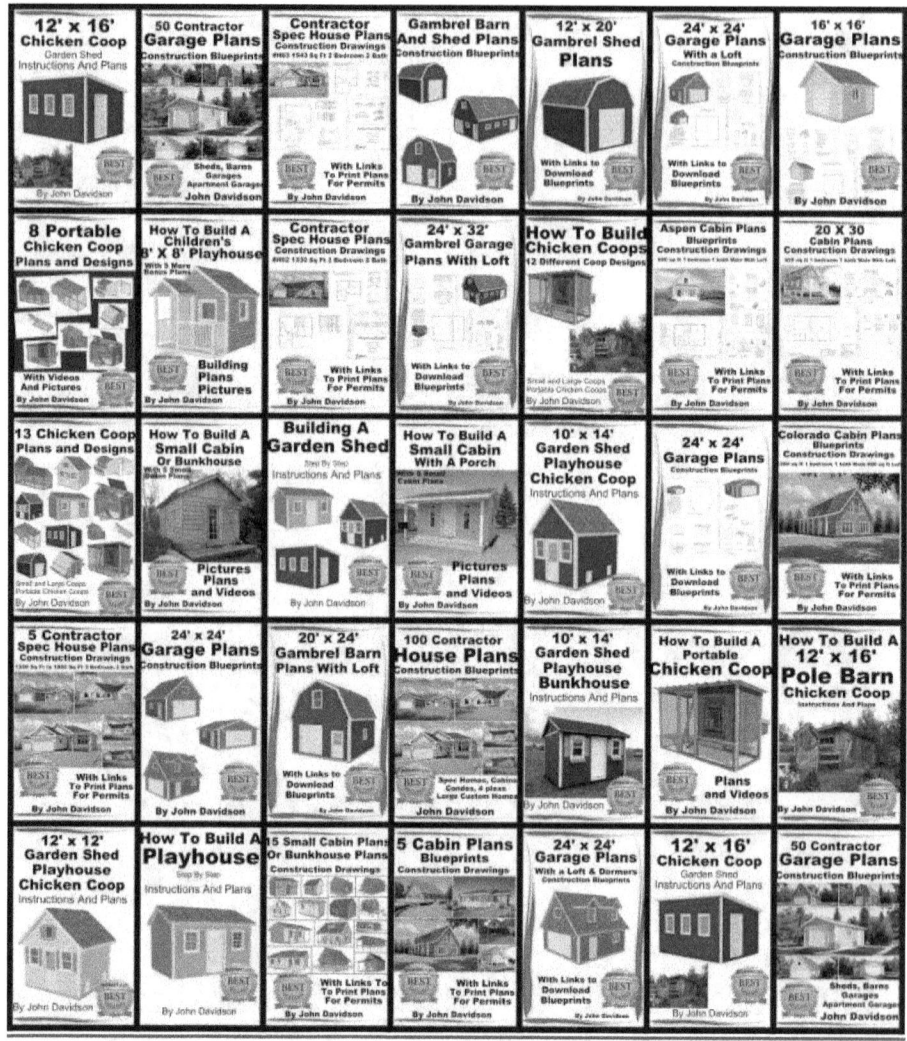

Entrepreneur Book Series

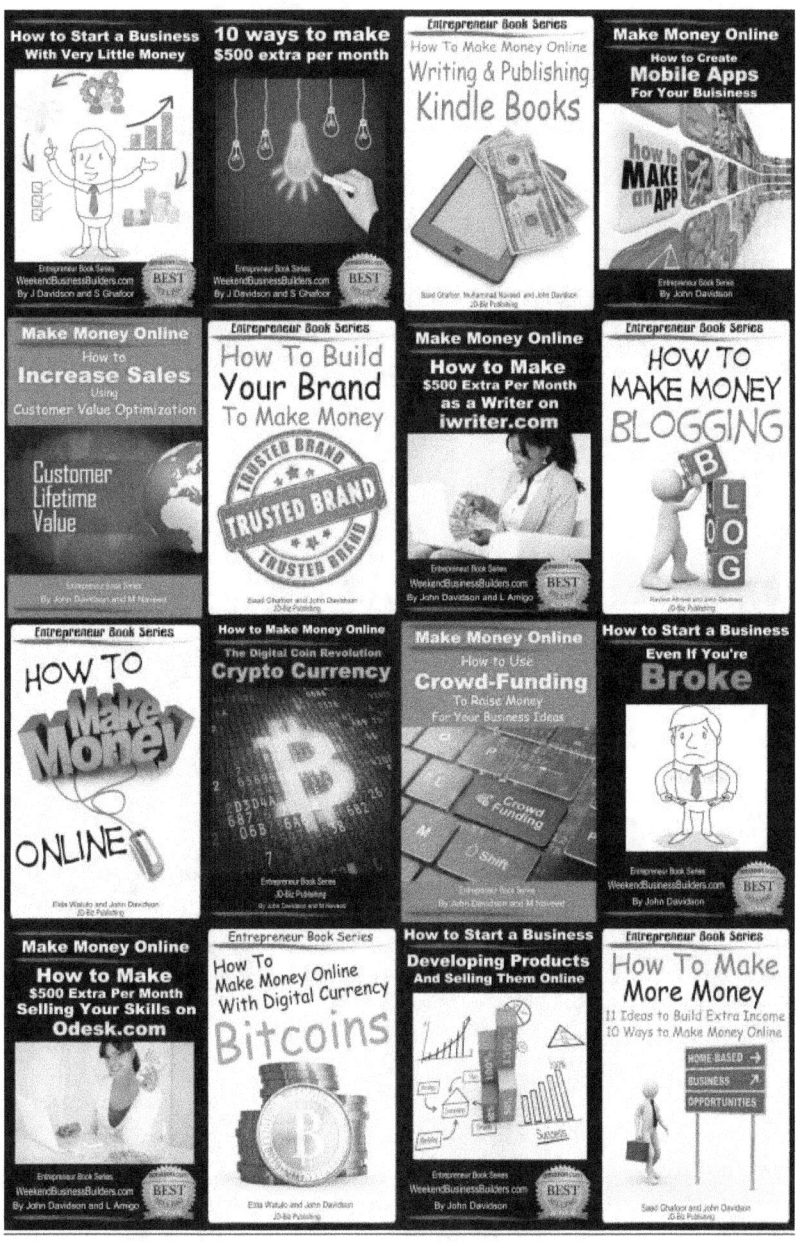

Our books are available at

1. Amazon.com

2. Barnes and Noble

3. Itunes

4. Kobo

5. Smashwords

6. Google Play Books

Publisher

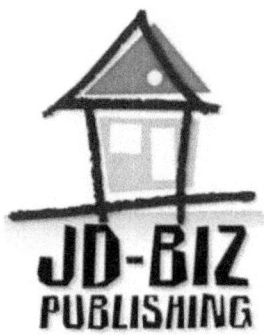

JD-Biz Corp

P O Box 374

Mendon, Utah 84325

http://www.jd-biz.com/

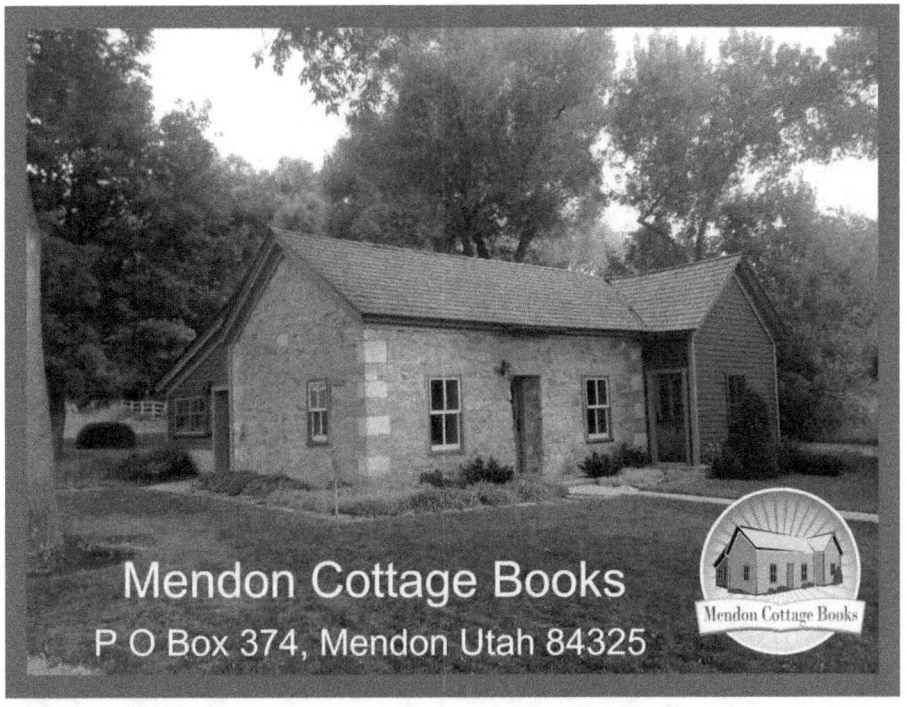